Dog Walking
Reflections Through the Seasons

Dog Walking

Reflections Through the Seasons

John Henry Reininger

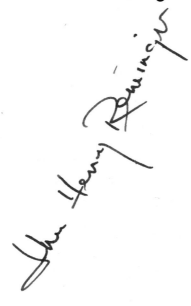

Dog Walking
Reflections Through the Seasons

by John Henry Reininger

ISBN: 978-0-9832485-2-1
Library of Congress Control Number: 2011901280

Book designed by Nehmen-Kodner: www.n-kcreative.com
Printed in the United States of America

Published by John Henry Reininger
dogwalkingreflections.com · john@dogwalkingreflections.com

Dedication

To my family and friends of both the
two- and four-legged varieties who live
in Ohio, in Florida and in my heart.

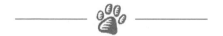

Contents

Acknowledgments

Any endeavor such as this does not happen in isolation. My love and most sincere appreciation for her constant support, encouragement, and wise input go to Ellen Moran Fraser. Without her this project would not have taken place. She was and continues to be my muse. The expertise of Mary Margaret Dolan's editing transformed many rough drafts into presentable text.

The dogs who have been my walking companions for many years have recently changed. Molly yielded her place for another rescue Sheltie, Katie, in February of 2009. She will be missed, but like all that have gone before her, Molly will always have a special place in my heart.

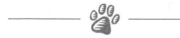

A portion of the sale from *Dog Walking*
will be donated to the following organizations:

Humane Society of Broward County
2070 Griffin Road
Fort Lauderdale, FL 33312

Shetland Sheepdog Rescue Fund
American Shetland Sheepdog Association
PO Box 819
New Lenox, IL 60451

Introduction

For more than twenty-five years as a licensed psychotherapist I have worked with people who were seeking ways to improve the quality of their lives. This book presents values and principles that many have found beneficial.

Dog Walking is a collection of observations. These stories originated while walking my Shelties around our suburban neighborhood. Each day I discover something that has the potential to enrich life.

In compiling this book two truths became evident. First, walking dogs is not necessary to fully embrace life. Second, being open to change is not always easy but is invariably rewarding.

It is my sincere hope that you find the stories inspiring. If you choose to do the exercises, you may find them helpful in unlocking the wonderful possibilities that reside in you each day.

Story Format

Each story has a singular focus and is complete at that point. If you wish to go further onto the topic, the subsequent headings can help you explore insights into your own life.

The book is divided into seasons. Throughout the year there are only subtle temperature changes in South Florida. What does vary is the emotional ebb and flow in the passing months. Our lives also have seasons. These are defined by time and experience. Seasons are about life.

The components of each narrative are:

1. The Experience
My observations as we walk around our neighborhood.

2. Walking Light
A brief reflection based on the story's theme.

3. Personal Path
This section encourages journaling. It is a technique with established therapeutic value. It can reinforce insight and change. Journal entries can be made in a notebook or on the computer.

There is also the opportunity to begin a minijournal at the end of this book.

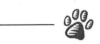

Summer

A life without love is like a year without summer.

—*Swedish Proverb*

The summer season is busy. It is a time for growth and work. It is a time to play and relax. What we choose to do in the summer needs to sustain us through the challenges that inevitably lay ahead.

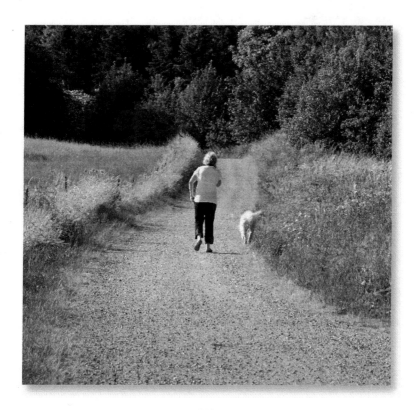

Sheepless

My walking companions are Molly and Calvin. They are Shetland sheepdogs, part of a herding breed, affectionately known as Shelties. Both are "rescued" dogs and as far as I know have never seen a herd of anything. Being in the outdoors for our walks is the only common link with their ancestors' lifestyle. Our walks, I believe, stir a deep yearning within them. Their natural environment is rural fields and flocks. The suburban streets of Fort Lauderdale are very different. Yet, they bounce and bark every time I put on their leashes.

The combination of fresh air and sunlight creates a sense of wellness found nowhere else. It fosters a sense of vibrancy to live better and love deeper. Sharing the experience of being outside makes it even more special.

The joy Molly and Calvin find in the outdoors, even without sheep, keeps them healthy. Spending time in our original natural environment still benefits us.

Reflection: Playtime

◆ Walking Light

Having fun is essential to a healthy lifestyle. As children we naturally discovered this through playtime. Often it was outside. Childhood play reduced stress and built social skills. In addition, such joyful experiences created lifetime memories.

As adults recreation can encompass a much wider selection of activities. The essential element is still finding a sense of fun in the process. When we interact with others who share the same feeling of joy, the whole positive experience is amplified.

◆ Personal Path

In your journal or notebook recall playtimes you had as a child outside. Next, look back over the past month and write down where you experienced a sense of fun. What portion of that was outdoors?

Love puts fun in together, sad in apart,
and joy in a heart.

—Anonymous

The Lizard Chaser and Mr. Cool

In South Florida small lizards are a common sight. At times Molly's primary objective is to chase, herd, and capture as many as possible. To date, her results in this endeavor equal zero. That statistical fact does not deter her. Calvin remains above these antics and ignores her. Although my dogs are the same breed, their personalities are quite different.

I appreciate the unique qualities of each dog. Too often in relationships one partner is trying to change the other. Acceptance is not considered. This damages both individuals and the potential of the relationship.

Reflection: Nurturing Relationships

+ **Walking Light**

Building a healthy relationship requires knowing and nurturing your own values. And it requires respecting your partner's values. Then we can enjoy the similarities and accept the differences of each.

+ **Personal Path**

Make a journal entry of a personal strength as well as one of your partner's. Next, write what you have done to nurture those in the past week.

Wherever you go, go with all your heart.

—Confucius

Cloud Topper

Some things happen in the blink of an eye and leave a permanent impression. The other morning presented such a happenstance. In the predawn sky, a long, vertical cloud was topped by the shape of the crescent moon. It only lasted for an instant and then was gone. I said "WOW" out loud with only the dogs to hear.

A streak of lightning disappears in fractions of a second. Yet, it leaves behind a strong mental image. A gentle touch, caring word, or warm smile requires very little time. These small kindnesses leave an impression as well.

A thoughtful gesture can create a timeless legacy. "Topping" someone's day may take only a little effort; however, in the end both giver and receiver benefit.

Molly and Calvin's walks are "topped" by a meal, a treat, or a good back scratching! They enjoy the experience. So do I!

Reflection: Small Kindnesses

◆ Walking Light

The power to change can be found in the littlest of kind acts. An expression of thoughtfulness enriches lives. It is as simple as saying "Hello" or "Thank You." Although it may only take a moment, the impact continues much longer.

◆ Personal Path

Write about a recent small kindness you received that "topped" your day. What made it meaningful for you?

No act of kindness, no matter how small, is ever wasted.

—*Aesop's* The Lion and the Mouse

Distance

I have never measured the distance we walk each day. The dogs and I are gaining in years both human and dog type. For certain the distance we travel has become shorter. Regardless, on each walk we encounter two types of distance. One is lineal, that is the streets we walk. The second is vertical, the universe above our heads.

Our lives also have vastly different dimensions. Busy and quiet, joyful and sad, close and isolated are components we experience. Sometimes these occur in quick succession. There is an instinctive need for balance. Too much of one and not enough of the other can be unsettling.

Slow, stop, fast, slow is the typical pace of our walks. Eventually we return home. Life seldom flows in perfect harmony. It is our individual responsibility to make time for renewal. Balance requires nurturing the dimensions of our spirit, body, and heart. When this happens we return "home" to an inner calm that creates strength for tomorrow.

Reflection: Balance

• **Walking Light**

When life is out of balance, complaints are numerous. To rebalance requires personal involvement. Persistence, creativity, and prayerfulness are components of that process. The time to start is today.

• **Personal Path**

The act of journaling requires both time and effort. You are worth it. Identify how you rebalanced life after an upsetting event. What did you do to accomplish this?

Life is like riding a bicycle. To keep your balance you must keep moving.

—Albert Einstein

Bulk Trash Pickup

They are like mini mountains temporarily appearing around the neighborhood. Each collection is comprised of yard waste, broken furniture, and a wide assortment of mysterious stuff. These spontaneous hills will disappear by the end of the day.

There is an instinct to hold onto the past. Often this is through photos, antiques, and certainly with memories. As we do, it adds a sense of personal depth. When acknowledging the past, we can gain insight to ourselves. Where we have been becomes a guide to where we want to go.

Molly and Calvin continue to move along looking for what is just ahead. They do not spend time reflecting on thoughts like "I should have done…!" They are dogs. Humans at times hold on to past regrets. Our challenge is to "sort through" past experiences. Discard what is not helpful. Then, it becomes possible to say "I can do…!"

Reflection: Heritage

✦ Walking Light

We are an accumulation of past experiences. This creates a heritage unique to each individual. It is each person's responsibility to select the parts to build on. This passes along a healthy heritage for the future.

✦ Personal Path

Locate old family photographs. In your journal write out memories you have of these individuals. How are you similar or different? What was their heritage to you?

In order to plan your future wisely, it is necessary that you understand and appreciate your past.

—Jo Coudert

Stains

The street surface is like a dark gray canvas. These roads record the passage of those who use them.

On any walk it is easy to see the traces of life. Here is where a car caught on fire. Over there are oil stains. Just beyond hunks of tar. Some have been around for years while others will disappear by the next day. Temporary or indelible the roadway records all.

The canvas of our life is tinted by each passing encounter. Some experiences leave a permanent mark. Others occur without causing much of an impression. It is important to assess how different events impact us.

I realized as we turned the last corner before home that the ordinary is not really ordinary. This is a new day to be filled with new experiences and leaving its own impressions.

Reflection: Perspective

◆ **Walking Light**

Each experience has an impact on our perspective. Some experiences have the power to change even long-held viewpoints. It is our challenge to be open to "see" alternative ideas and then keep or change our position.

◆ **Personal Path**

Write in your journal about a recent event that changed your perspective.

What we see depends on mainly what we look for.

—John Lubbock

Taxi

At first I was not certain what I saw in the distance. As Molly, Calvin, and I drew closer, it became distinct. An older man had attached a small canvas-covered trailer to the rear axle of his bicycle. Inside was his dog, enjoying the ride. I suspect this "taxi" service was necessary because his dog could no longer take extended walks outside. The compassion this elderly man expressed towards his beloved companion still allowed them to spend time together.

Life changes us. Physical transitions occur over the years. Activities once mutually shared with someone special may no longer be possible. There is one factor that does not need to change, treasuring time together.

I no longer see the pair. What does remain with me is this: the compassion for his companion and the pleasure of that friendship go well beyond their ride together.

Reflection: Compassion

◆ Walking Light

There is a difference between feeling sorry for someone and having compassion for that person. You can feel sorry for someone and not be involved in his or her life. Compassion is care put into action.

◆ Personal Path

Write about a time you showed true compassion to someone.

*I would rather feel compassion
than know the meaning of it.*

—Thomas Aquinas

Floating Lights

During the summer months the tropical foliage becomes even denser. The street's lights struggle to illuminate beyond the immediate wreaths of surrounding leaves. In the darkness it is easy to see the light, but the supporting pole is invisible as if it were suspended in midair.

Experiencing depression is similar. We can feel the depression but can't identify what is feeding it. Asking ourselves "why" has the potential of only darkening the mood. "What can I do?" begins the process of easing depression's burden.

The darkness of early morning slowly yields to first light as we head towards home. Working through the blackness of depression allows the warm light of life to shine through.

Reflection: Emotional Well-being

+ **Walking Light**

Depression, frustration, and anger can overwhelm us. Acknowledging these emotions takes courage. Once we do this, the path to emotional well-being becomes illuminated.

+ **Personal Path**

In your journal identify an emotionally trying time or situation. What did you do to regain a sense of well-being?

Depression is the inability to construct a future.

—Rollo May

Sidewalk Patterns

In South Florida the soil is very sandy. Yard sprinklers often wash the sand across the bordering concrete sidewalks. This morning I noticed a pattern of water-carved sand on the walkway. What was just a flat plain surface yesterday is now embossed.

Creativity needs a solid base upon which to be expressed. An artist uses a canvas. In life our core values or strengths give us a foundation upon which we define ourselves. This clarity of values then allows for the assertive expression of creativity.

We finish our walk just at daybreak. As we move through the day our core values remain constant. And then our creative mind builds upon those values.

Reflection: Core Values

◆ **Walking Light**

Core values provide a framework for life. Within that framework qualities such as integrity, respect, compassion, tolerance, spirituality, and others develop. We flourish as these are put into action.

◆ **Personal Path**

Write about the values you brought from your childhood. How have they been used in your adult life?

*Open your arms to change
but don't let go of your values.*

—Dalai Lama

Fast Walks

Nearby lightning and torrential rain make for hasty outings. Regardless of the weather Molly and Calvin start with equal enthusiasm. At such times my motivation is different.

Each day is also the beginning of our "walk" through the coming hours. Sometimes we are faced with so much to do and very little time to accomplish it. Such days seem to go by quickly. Yet, the same number of hours exist when "time drags." The difference is waiting or being involved.

In life we can choose to be an observer or participant. The irony is when we are active and participate, more possibilities can be found in the "shorter day."

Reflection: Possibilities

• **Walking Light**

Each day has possibilities. Each of us has the ability to access these possibilities. To learn, to grow, to give, to forgive, to do, are only a few. It is a personal decision to reach out and "grab" them.

• **Personal Path**

Possibilities can be found through daily tasks. In your journal, write about an ordinary chore at work or home. What did you do after completion of this task? Therein are found possibilities.

We all are gifted. That is our inheritance.

—Ethel Waters

Senses

Senses become heightened when I walk the dogs during darkness. Sight is limited, but sound and smell are sharpened. How Molly and Calvin react at these times is unknown. For myself, the sound of a car approaching from behind us has my acute attention. The lingering aroma of a barbecue certainly is pleasant. Even the murmur of the neighbor's water fountain seems more prominent.

There are times that certain emotions such as sadness and depression are stronger. It changes how we experience even each moment. The comfortable flow of an ordinary day becomes difficult. What was familiar now feels strange. Our responsibility is not to ignore these feelings but to work through them.

At night the darkness remains for the entire walk. The brightness and comfort of our home awaits a few blocks away. It feels good to be there again.

Reflection: Awareness

◆ Walking Light

A truly enriched life is one where our senses and emotions are engaged. Such awareness does not come from being hurried. Stop. Look. Listen. Breathe. Touch. Feel. Honoring God's creation of the universe that surrounds us comes through using all our senses.

◆ Personal Path

We can become more aware of how our senses enrich our life. Write something you observe about each of the five senses—sight, hearing, smell, touch, and taste.

There is a way that nature speaks, that land speaks. Most of the time we are simply not patient enough, quiet enough to pay attention to the story.

—Linda Hogan

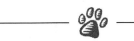

Autumn

There is a harmony in autumn and a luster in the sky,
which through the summer is not heard or seen,
as if it could not be, as if it had not been!

—Percy Bysshe Shelly

In the fall of life we celebrate and acknowledge all that has been accomplished. It is a transitional time, a bridge between past and future. In autumn we focus on gathering and thankfulness.

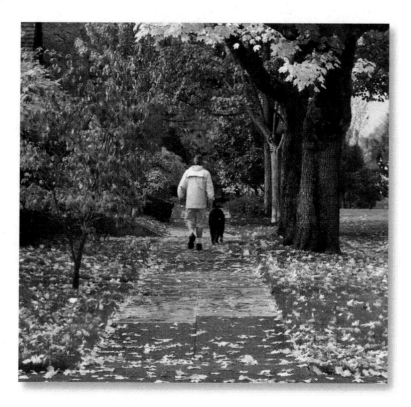

Half-Staffed

Every generation has one. Ours is 9/11. Around the neighborhood this September morning the American flag is flown at half staff. It is a silent tribute to an unimaginable event. As Molly, Calvin, and I walked by each flag I said a silent prayer. It was for those who died this day. The prayer was also for the generations yet to come whose lives have been irrevocably changed.

Emotions and events connect us. We are quiet passing strangers to those houses. We are also connected because of a commonly shared event. As individuals we have the power to isolate or join with others. It is a power to be used wisely.

Reflection: Connectedness

Walking Light

How we connect to others changes as we grow. Grade school friends, high school coaches, the first girlfriend or boyfriend all mark our emotional and cognitive development. Continued healthy interactions build quality connections that carry us into the future.

Personal Path

In your journal, write about a special person who helped form who you are today.

Only through our connectedness to others
can we really know and enhance the self.
And only through working on the self can we begin
to enhance our connectedness to others.

—Harriet Goldhor Lerner

Things That Go Bump In The Night

We walk in moonlight more than in sunlight. The streets are quiet. The trees, bushes, and yards are still. Every so often the quietness is suddenly broken by rustling sounds from inside the nearby foliage. It is always surprising and a little unsettling. If I have been lulled into peaceful thoughts they immediately end. Emotions take over. Sometimes the dogs are alert to the noise. Most often they ignore it.

Surprises can be fun as well as unpleasant. Reacting to both is natural. When something traumatic occurs strong emotions can be stirred. These are not to be ignored. It takes courage to work through them. In doing so, you begin to regain control of your well-being.

We finish our walk and return safely home again. When difficulties and the corresponding feelings are confronted, we can create a quiet courage that carries us through each day.

Reflection: Courage

♦ Walking Light

Being courageous can happen every day. It is not easy to stand by your values when others want you to compromise them. Yet, as we show courage, life can begin to attain a steadfast quality.

♦ Personal Path

Write in your journal about decisions you have made that took courage.

All serious daring starts from within.

—Harriet Beecher Stowe

Seamless

Our neighborhood was developed in the early 1970s. At the time the roads were paved first on one side then the other. The seam between each half now is only noticeable due to a slightly different tint on the road's surface. The street itself is smooth where it joins together.

One day seamlessly follows the next. Most often the transition flows smoothly. Yet, each day does have its own characteristics. The challenges we find along the way can build confidence in facing an unknown tomorrow. This ability comes through our successes and mistakes.

Molly, Calvin, and I walk on these streets with familiar ease each day. We know them well. Be confident. This helps make life's journey easier.

Reflection: Confidence

+ **Walking Light**

Effort is required to transform natural abilities into skills. These in turn give us confidence to make the most of each day. It is important to give yourself credit for accomplishments.

+ **Personal Path**

Confidence results from a process of accumulation. It is built on achievements small and large. Describe in your journal those areas in which you feel confident.

You have to have confidence in your ability and then be tough enough to follow through.

—Rosalyn Carter

And Then There Were Three—Almost

S ome time ago I believed that walking three dogs would be not much more of a challenge than two. To follow through on this hunch I went "sightseeing" at the local Humane Society. Temptation is hard to resist. On an early November day I met "Holly" at the shelter. I am not certain who spotted who first. Cleverly, this large Belgium Shepherd did everything possible to say, "Take me home, PLEASE!" She was a great salesperson!

The staff did all the necessary paperwork to begin the adoption process. Much to my disappointment they found the zoning code in the area where I lived allowed only two dogs per household. I am not certain who was more let down—Holly or me.

Setbacks are part of life. They happen sometimes when we dare to dream. Life would be much poorer if we did not dream.

My hope is that Holly found a loving home. Personal dreams, even unfulfilled, find their own special place in memories.

Reflection: Dreams

+ **Walking Light**

Dreams are where future goals begin to form. If we hold on to too many disappointments we become afraid to dream. Simply thinking "what if..." in a positive way is the beginning of a dream. Allow it to unfold.

+ **Personal Path**

Write about something for which you wished. What did you do in trying to fulfill this wish or dream?

Nothing happens unless we dream.

—Carl Sandburg

Colors

The transition from summer to fall is different in South Florida. In other climates foliage changes to tones of reds and gold. Here the colors of out-of-state license plates become more dominant. Every year northern automobiles and their occupants head south for the warm weather by late October.

While ice crystals add sparkle to bare branches up north, orange Halloween lights brighten palm trees around the neighborhood. Vibrant-hued flowers begin to flourish here while colors in the north slip into shades of brown and gray.

Life is filled with transitions in health, living styles, and beliefs. How we move in and out of them will vary. We do know that change is certain.

Reflection: Transitions

+ **Walking Light**

Transitions in life can happen in a moment or take a year. They can be challenging or flow easily. Although you may have limited influence over the transition, the impact is another matter. Regardless of what happened you can choose to grow as a result.

+ **Personal Path**

Write about a recent event that changed from the original plans. What was the impact on you both in the short and long term?

Not in his goals but in his transitions is man great.

—*Ralph Waldo Emerson*

Wet Feet

It was a group of three. An elderly man, a young boy, and an even younger puppy were walking together in the early morning light. A light rain shower had just stopped. As we passed each other the youngster shared his worry about his little dog getting wet feet. With a gentle reassurance from the senior member of the entourage, the young fellow returned to happily chatting.

The best gift to a relationship is to be yourself. The mutual sharing of thoughts and feelings makes this possible.

The elderly gentleman and child experienced the same stroll from different perspectives. Being able to express our uniqueness is essential. "Editing" such expression restricts the potential of a relationship.

Reflection: Uniqueness

◆ Walking Light

Like snowflakes, there are no two humans exactly alike. Honoring those unique qualities in yourself is essential. Habits change through the course of our lives. Who we are does not change.

◆ Personal Path

In your journal, identify those situations where it is difficult to express your thoughts or emotions. Next write what you would like to say.

Never apologize for showing feelings.
When you do so, you apologize for the truth.

—Benjamin Disraeli

Bells and Whistles

It is not uncommon to meet another dog walker on our rounds. Last night at dusk this occurred but there was a difference. In addition to walking her pooch, she was reading a book with a small attached portable light, and using a hands-free cell phone at the same time. The dog was wearing an orange safety vest with a small blinking red light on its collar. The simple task of walking her dog became complex.

How often in life do we make something simple more complicated? Too often we add distractions. It takes a conscious effort to remain on the original course of action.

I wondered if this dog walker was giving quality attention to any of her activities. Fortunately traffic was light on our street. To keep things simple it is best to focus on one task at a time.

Reflection: Simplicity

+ **Walking Light**

There are many aspects to any task. But even the most involved pro-
cedure is done one step at a time. The challenge is to do each part to
the best of our ability. Then we can feel a sense of pride in what was
accomplished.

+ **Personal Path**

In a short sentence identify one simple thing you enjoy doing each
day.

Simply the thing that I am shall make me live.

—William Shakespeare

Blink

Near the edge of where Molly, Calvin, and I walk is a stop light. At 5:30AM this traffic signal is in blink mode. Drivers need to trust that opposing cars will either slow on the yellow side or stop on the red light side. If ignored, the consequences can be tragic.

Trusting someone you know is easy. Trusting a stranger is another matter. When trust is broken it takes a conscious effort on both sides to rebuild. What happens carelessly can require years to reestablish. Only when those involved are willing to be hurt again can trust be renewed.

By the time we finish our walk the traffic light has returned to its normal cycle. Cars proceed through the intersection as they have done for years without incident. I also continue my day placing trust in God watching over me. That protection has never failed.

Reflection: Trust

✦ Walking Light

Trust builds growth. Relationships flourish. Ultimately, trusting is a gift of honest love. It is based upon words and deeds matching. It is where behaviors often speak louder than those words.

✦ Personal Path

Journal about an experience where it was important to trust someone.

Without trust words become the hollow sound of a wooden gong. With trust words become life.

—Anonymous

Two Trees

In the decades since our neighborhood was developed many lush and large trees have grown. They are familiar landmarks that add a visual quality to our walks. Yesterday morning a tree company removed two large pines from a side yard. Now an open starkness exists where once there was shade. The landscape once enriched by the trees was now empty.

The trees had a finite value. A car, clothing, computer also have value found in their use. The laughter of a child, a lover's touch, a long friendship has intrinsic value beyond count. Recognizing true wealth is to be aware of life's intangible elements.

My canine companions certainly provide a quality to life not otherwise attainable. I believe I add to their well-being. Their abundant tail wagging may be a good indicator of this fact. The end result: all our lives are enhanced.

Reflection: True Wealth

♦ Walking Light

Family and friends are the "currency" that gives our life true wealth.
It is a richness that not only enhances each day but extends to time's
end. The true quality of this "wealth" is established through caring
interactions with those about us.

♦ Personal Path

In your journal make a brief inventory of your most valued possessions. Next make a list of the three people who are most important
in your life today. Which list has the highest "value"?

Our true wealth is the good we do in this world.
None of us has faith unless we desire for our neighbors
what we desire for ourselves.

—Mohammed

Wind Chimes

There are a number of wind chimes underneath the eaves of a house along our route. On a typical day they produce an almost whimsical sound. This morning in the still air there was only silence. It felt unnatural as the chimes' musical potential was left unfulfilled.

Each of us has potential. The "winds" of opportunity stir that potential every day. Unlike the chimes, we can choose to act. We can also choose to be still. When we decide to do even the smallest of tasks, the "music" of accomplishment happens. In using the God-given talents we all possess, life becomes a symphony.

In the evening a breeze picked up. As we passed by, the tones of the metal and glass shapes once again came alive. Molly and Calvin paid no attention. How much we are "in tune" with life is important.

Reflection: Potential

✦ Walking Light

Your potential is a renewable resource. It is inertia waiting to be used. The more you exercise your creative potential, the more expansive life becomes and the more others are impacted. Think. Create. Move.

✦ Personal Path

Realizing potential starts with an open mind and heart. Write about a time when negative thinking kept you from exploring a new direction.

It is the creative potential itself in human beings that is the image of God.

—Mary Daly

A Familiar Song

The ritual is simple. In late fall, before our predawn walk, I open the front door to see if a sweater is needed. This morning in doing this I heard a distant car radio. It was playing a catchy familiar song. Although lasting only a few seconds the melody played repeatedly in my head throughout the walk.

Prayers can be like a familiar song. There is comfort in recalling them. Regardless of whether they are from childhood or new, they touch a deep spiritual chord within us. It is an intrinsic yearning for solace, hope, or renewal attainable in no other way.

After a while the words of a popular song can "wear thin." The opposite happens with prayers. They gain a luster with use and age.

Reflection: Prayer

◆ Walking Light

The "melody" of familiar prayers is a connection. In prayer we are reaching into a special time and place and ultimately, eternity. Spirituality is fostered through prayer. It is a unique source of strength. When all else has been tried on our human level, we turn to prayer.

As children, we may have prayed primarily at bedtime or at meals. Now, as adults we can pray anytime. Prayer is not based on skill but on a heartfelt belief. And in that belief we discover God.

◆ Personal Path

In your journal compose a simple prayer. Reflect on it from time to time.

In prayer it is better to have a heart without words than words without heart.

—Mahatma Gandhi

Strays

There is a leash law in our neighborhood. As Molly, Calvin, and I make our circuit, occasionally a loose dog suddenly appears. My canine companions recognize a relative and bark. I react differently. The intentions of this stray visitor are unknown. I am deciding what to do next.

When the unexpected occurs a number of possibilities can follow. Choosing to respond in the best way possible determines the quality of what happens next. The challenge is making the decision with the information at hand. A healthy choice is not always the easiest one.

We continued our walk. I said strong words of encouragement for the stray to do the same. The entire encounter took less than a minute. Regardless, an important lesson was learned. In life I can be active and make decisions or passive and be victim to circumstances. I choose the former.

Reflection: Healthy Choices

• Walking Light

Making healthy choices requires making clear and timely decisions. Regardless of whether the decision is spur-of-the-moment or planned, a healthy decision respects all who are involved.

• Personal Path

In your journal write about a decision you made that you felt was a good one. It could be as simple as a healthy meal or as complex as a lifestyle change.

What we call the secret of happiness is no more a secret than our own willingness to choose life.

—Leo Buscaglia

Moving Day

Large moving vans are temporary obstacles that we walk around. These metallic whales hold a family's treasures. Regardless of whether they are moving away or just relocating to the area, changes in that family's life are taking place.

Relocation is part of life. We have been doing it since childhood. Changing classrooms, transferring from one job to the next, and moving in with a girlfriend or boyfriend are ways we relocate. If we move to improve life, prosperity can follow. A long-term positive outcome is more difficult if we are running away.

Molly, Calvin, and I continue to pass by the moving truck. As the activity continues, I hope that optimism is part of that family's possessions.

Reflection: Optimism

◆ Walking Light

Optimism is a value that helps us discover the best in ourselves. We need to "unpack" and discard some of the negative thinking that limits our outlook. Holding on to words such as "I can't" only restricts. Saying "I'll give it a try" helps promote optimism.

◆ Personal Path

Watch the news for a day. Write down the stories that impressed you. Were they about overcoming some difficulty? What part did optimism play in achieving the end result?

It's not that optimism solves all of life's problems; it is just that it can sometimes make the difference between coping and collapsing.

—Lucy Macdonald

Daylight

Street lights have a simple function—to illuminate. They are either on or off. When it is dark they provide a safer passage for us and the cars. On our lunchtime walk I noticed one of the lights remained on, despite the bright sunlight. Apparently the automatic sensor that switches it off was stuck. Only a dull glare was evident from the bulb serving no practical purpose.

Habits, routines, and skills help us navigate through each day. They provide coping skills. However, times can occur when we get "stuck." Our established resources are not enough to meet the new challenge. Only by considering a different approach do we increase the probability to resolve the issue and move on.

Molly, Calvin, and I pass beneath the stuck light. It has no choice but to remain lit. When we find ourselves trapped, we do have a choice to change. Making such a decision gets us unstuck.

Reflection: Getting Unstuck

✦ Walking Light

Habits are like old friends; they are familiar. Overall they have helped us through to this day. Good habits enable us to continue moving forward and restrictive ones hold us back. It is these latter habits that get us stuck.

✦ Personal Path

Write about a habit that you have changed. What was your motivation? What is the difference in your life now?

Don't wish it was easier; wish you were better.
Don't wish for less problems; wish for more skills.
Don't wish for less challenges; wish for more wisdom.

—Jim Rohn

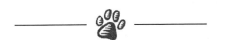

Winter

Winter must be cold for those with no warm memories.

—*Movie:* An Affair to Remember

Reflection on the important elements in your life can reinforce a sense of comfort. Winter provides such a time. Reflect to "recharge" before moving towards the coming renewal.

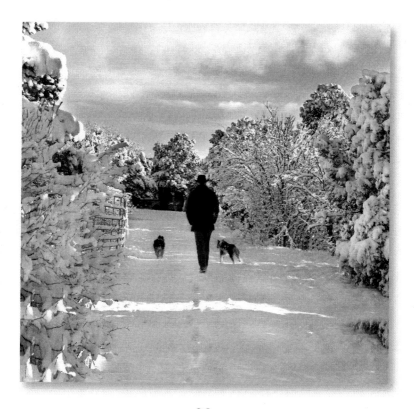

Dog Ears

A pickup truck drove past us yesterday during our midday walk. The side windows were open to the cool winter air. Out of those windows were the heads of two enthusiastic dogs—a brown Boxer and a black Lab. The truck cab as a result looked like it had a set of large ears!

As they went by, the dogs were constantly changing places from one side to the other. This canine coordination gave them a total view. I was amazed how easily they switched without apparent disagreement.

When working together, much can be accomplished.

Reflection: Cooperation

+ **Walking Light**

Teams depend on the individual skill of each participant. Cooperation between all members then achieves goals not otherwise possible. Volunteer to be part of a team effort at home, school, or in your community. It takes many hands to build bridges.

+ **Personal Path**

In your journal write out the following: 1. Identify a situation where you helped another attain his or her goal. 2. How did this impact you?

Two heads are better than one.

—Polish Proverb

Going Outside

Molly and Calvin are "inside" dogs. When we are about to take a walk, their individual reactions are quite different. Molly bounces about at first and then stands waiting for her leash. Calvin just sits patiently.

Life presents us with events that will challenge the patience of some while others take it in stride. It is important to recognize what you can and cannot do in each situation. If there is no choice in changing the external circumstances, then choose to change how you handle it internally. Impatience is exhausting, and it will wear you down.

Our walk is finished and I prepare breakfast for my companions, a reward for their patience.

Reflection: Patience

◆ Walking Light

Being patient in situations that you control is seldom difficult. Our patience is tested when we are not in control. You can develop patience by taking personal responsibility to deescalate the internal stress reactions.

◆ Personal Path

Describe in your journal something that requires your patience. What makes it easy or difficult to express patience in that situation?

Patience is the companion to wisdom.

—St. Augustine

Night

There is a short part of our route that changes dramatically at night. It has no street lights and the road is covered by a heavy canopy of trees. In the darkness it is difficult to see where the pavement ends and the grassy swale begins. The horizon and sky are hidden. It is all very black.

Sadness and loss are emotional darkness. They mute the vibrant colors of life. Uncertainty is dominant. The future is difficult to see.

Molly, Calvin, and I pass through this area in a minute or two. We keep moving and once again reach the lit street just ahead. Grief is a process that also requires movement. It takes an inordinate amount of strength to reengage with life. The effort is worth it.

Reflection: Living Through Loss

◆ **Walking Light**
Part of life is loss. The strength to work through the grief is found in good self-care, a deep respect for the quality of life, and a belief in the future.

◆ **Personal Path**
Write about a loss you experienced. This can be a relationship, job, death, or health issue. How did you change as a result?

Death leaves a heartache no one can heal,
love leaves a memory no one can steal.

—From a headstone in Ireland

Dry

The winter months are dry in South Florida. This past season was exceptionally parched. Our natural water supply was critically low, so municipalities restricted lawn watering and car washing. The green lawns along our walk began to turn brown while the owners were turning red. Water conservation was becoming defined more by tension than benefit. There were still the defiant owners who were sprinkling their grass every day.

Sometimes our focus is short and selfish. The needs for our own gratification overshadow a larger common good. Conservation is more than just "going green." It is the appreciation of God's creation put into action.

Reflection: Conservation

+ **Walking Light**

Conservation applies to the world about us and ourselves as well. We are not indestructible nor do we have limitless strength. To be our best we need to be good managers of our personal resources. A balanced physical, emotional, and spiritual pace nourishes life.

+ **Personal Path**

In your journal record the actions you take to conserve both the environment and yourself.

We do not inherit the earth from our ancestors;
we borrow it from our children.

—*Native American Proverb*

Office Neighborhood Friend

I am able to bring Molly and Calvin to my office. The bordering neighborhood has its own population of canine inhabitants. One morning we met one of them. Running unleashed ahead of his human companion was Max. He was twice the size of my Shelties. With a shaggy brown coat and friendly personality he became the goodwill ambassador to our area. It always was a pleasure to see him running about.

Several years have passed since we have seen Max. His joyful disposition still brings warm memories. There was one thing about Max that became less obvious after many encounters. He was rescued from a terrible accident where he lost his right front leg.

Events happen in life that can become crippling. Our lives can be changed. Such changes can be crushing or evolutionary. That impact is up to the individual. Joy is not found in the event but in the nature of recovery.

I do not know what Max was like before we met. I do remember the joyful legacy he left. Perhaps he knew this secret: being involved with life is a joy.

Reflection: Joy

◆ **Walking Light**

Laughter is good medicine and joy its echo. When joy is shared it makes the difficult more bearable. And like any emotion it is found in various levels of intensity. Recognizing a quiet inner peace or laughing heartily is joy revealed.

◆ **Personal Path**

Find several photos of yourself smiling. Next find pictures from newspapers, magazines, cartoon, and so forth where happiness is evident. Place them in your journal with a comment on what you feel when looking at them. Remember that joy is all around but we need to invite it into our lives.

Joy is not on things, it is in us.

—*Richard Wagner*

Trees On Wheels

Immediately after Thanksgiving we see this annual phenomenon during our walks. A family car passes by with a Christmas tree firmly attached to the roof. Soon it will be decorated with child-made paper ornaments alongside delicate glass globes. There is also a bit of magic that happens in the transition. Individuals come together as family. They are united with a singular task to unpack memories and traditions. A special connection is once again renewed.

As the car with tree attached turns the corner, memories of my rural childhood come to mind. Family activities build a bridge connecting one generation to the next. It is our responsibility to make that span a sturdy one. The effort is worth it.

Reflection: Family

+ **Walking Light**

Gathering as family and friends has a unique power. We develop both individuality and corporate identities. In turn we are then connected to a larger entity—humankind.

+ **Personal Path**

In your journal record family traditions that were important in the past and still are part of your life today. These can be associated with a special event or as common as a weekly meal.

If the family were a fruit it would be an orange,
a circle of sections held together but separate—
each segment distinct.

—*Letty Cottin Pogrebin*

Curbside

"Silent Night" is now silent. Gifts have been opened and ornaments put away. It is mid-January. The once noble Christmas tree is now brown and brittle lying at the curbside. But remaining among those branches and in the stored boxes are memories of the past holiday season.

As we walk by this family's tree I hope it was a witness to much joy and gratitude. Heartfelt traditions would not exist without these elements.

There among the branches a delicate shimmering thread of silver tinsel glistened in the early morning light. It is like God's love woven through our lives every day. Even when we are down it is there to sustain us. We need to pause just briefly to recognize its comforting presence and then continue on our way.

Reflection: Gratitude

+ **Walking Light**

We can express gratitude in many ways each day through what we say and do. It fosters both warm interactions and cherished memories. It changes lives. It helps us grow. It gives us resilience.

+ **Personal Path**

In your journal recall instances where you said "thank you" today. Next write out the number of times you were thanked. Which was more frequent?

To speak gratitude is courteous and pleasant,
to enact gratitude is generous and noble,
but to live gratitude is to touch heaven.

—Johannes A. Gaertner

The Biscuit Lady

In all the years we have walked around our neighborhood this only happened once. What occurred left an indelible impression. One evening an elderly woman was slowly walking toward us. When we were about to pass one another she softly said "Hello." Then she asked if she could give Molly and Calvin a little treat. Of course my canine companions heard that genetically encoded word for food and responded with enthusiasm. Each received a dog biscuit.

Friendship begins by giving of oneself. When it is done without expectations the giver receives more in return than what was shared.

Reflection: Giving

◆ **Walking Light**

The best gifts come from the heart, not from the mall. The only cost incurred is caring. The value received exceeds the cost. And the best part is that one size fits all. Giving often is renewing.

◆ **Personal Path**

Write in your journal where you gave care today. How did you feel afterwards?

No one ever becomes poor by giving.

—Anne Frank

Hold On Tight

Yesterday evening another dog walker and I were about to pass by each other. From a distance her dog spotted us and began to bark. What she did next was unexpected. She picked up her small dog. Molly and Calvin remained silent while even by the end of the block her little dog was still barking.

Identifying and solving problems can be uniquely individual. Personal creativity is needed to develop effective coping skills.

This lady solved what she felt was an uncomfortable situation in the best way she knew. By her taking responsibility, we all continued along our journeys.

Reflection: Problem Solving

✦ Walking Light

At first the best solution to a problem may not be evident. Avoidance is seldom the optimum choice. This usually guarantees the return of the same issue. Even a small action directed towards a possible solution will make the next step more evident.

✦ Personal Path

What initial step did you take towards resolving a personal problem? Put this observation in your journal.

Problems are to the mind what exercise is to muscle, they toughen and make strong.

—Norman Vincent Peale

Passages

Black and gray outlines evolve into a multicolored landscape. This is what I see walking the dogs every morning. It is a natural passage of the earth to move from the darkness of night to the sunlit morning.

The passage from a single lifestyle into a relationship is a natural progression also. Both individuals bring their own unique qualities to that moment. These in turn amplify the singular identity of the friendship they create together.

At the end of our walk the neighborhood can be seen clearly, but it takes time for this to happen. The emotional tone of a relationship becomes more evident with time. Only with the contribution of two individuals, does it become filled with the warm glow of love.

Reflection: Identity

✦ Walking Light

We wear many "hats" during the course of a day. Parent, professional, friend, cook, and lover are just a few. All of these can be taken from you, for they are what we do. The only one that cannot be taken is who you are. It is internal. Surrendering it is the ultimate loss.

✦ Personal Path

How would you describe yourself? Warm, reserved, outgoing, strong-willed, spiritual, and considerate are some examples. Write about where this identity is most important in your life.

First say to yourself what would you be;
and then do what you have to.

—Epictetus

Spring

The day the Lord created hope was probably
the same day he created spring.

—Anonymous

At first there is a tentative subtleness to spring. We don't know the full possibilities ahead but have the sense of a positive future. Adapting to a renewed world requires believing in yourself and building towards the hope of a grand yet unknown tomorrow.

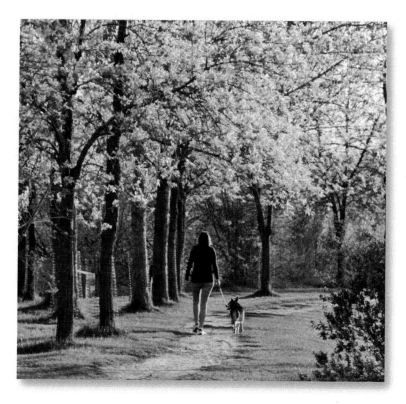

Shooting Stars

We live on the flight path of the local executive airport. Private aircraft are coming and going at all hours. With landing lights aglow, these fast-moving objects are like mechanical shooting stars. Instinctively I look at the airship flying overhead while Molly and Calvin are looking at the next clump of bushes. We have different interests and priorities.

Each day contains its own unique set of priorities. Some are familiar. Others are new. Either way, both require action.

Eventually the corporate jet will land. Its occupants will pursue the various priorities of business. The "business" of life sets before us choices. Our responsibility is to determine what is important and proceed accordingly.

Reflection: Prioritizing

+ **Walking Light**
The first step in completing any task is the most important. It may also be the most difficult. Attaining any goal greatly depends on a specific beginning point.

+ **Personal Path**
Write about a challenging project that you recently completed. Apply that same sense of accomplishment towards beginning the next task.

The key is not to prioritize what's on your schedule, but to schedule your priorities.

—Stephen Covey

Runner

Calvin's ears perked up and then he looked behind us. At that point I heard the footsteps of someone quickly approaching. It was an early morning runner. Passing us she said a brief "Good Morning!" Over the years joggers have been part of the sparse pedestrian traffic in the pre-dawn hours. These individuals really believe in the benefits of exercise.

Staying physically fit requires dedication. Cardio workouts or walking a few extra steps from a parking lot can be of benefit. Routinely exercising is nurturing both mentally and spiritually.

The walks Molly, Calvin, and I do may be considered marginal physical exercise. It is something more than I would probably do on my own. At times we need a little extra "nudge" to take good care of our bodies. The benefits of exercise pay dividends towards a healthier future.

Reflection: Exercise

◆ Walking Light

Physical exercise is more than walking from the TV or computer to the refrigerator! As children we channeled our energy into an active physical playtime. It often wore us out. We slept well and were happy. As adults the same principle holds true.

◆ Personal Path

In your journal make a commitment to yourself. Plan a conservative schedule of physical activity. Set a specific time to begin. You are worth the effort.

A man's health can be judged by which he takes
two at a time—pills or stairs.

—Joan Welsh·

Stars in Puddles

The spring in South Florida includes an ample number of rain showers. During our walks puddles are abundant. Last evening just after a rather heavy downpour there was a break in the overcast. I noticed the stars were reflected dimly in the standing water as we walked by.

When a loved one dies what remains is only a reflection of that life. The photos, personal possessions, even memories are merely an echo. There is no one to interact with, hold, or touch. We move into the storm of unknown grief. What's ahead seems unbearably dark.

After Molly and Calvin splash through the water fracturing the tiny points of starlight, the surface becomes calm once again. So it is with mourning. After we have worked through the emotional upheaval calmness returns to life. Then the memories become a reminder of the love that remains.

Reflection: Mourning

✦ Walking Light

Mourning is the emotional acknowledgment of an attachment that has changed. Its intensity is measured by the bond with the deceased. To focus on living requires realignment of both personal behaviors and the remaining emotional connections.

✦ Personal Path

"Marinating" in loss is not healthy. Moving ahead can require an extraordinary effort. Write about a loss and what you learned about yourself as a result.

A human life is a story told by God.

—*Hans Christian Anderson*

Mailbox

Most houses along our route have a mailbox attached to the front wall of the residence. This simple container opens a connection to the world beyond our street.

We have a special container within us—our soul. It is this spiritual essence that reaches beyond our daily lives into eternity. The grace of God gives us the strength to endure, to love, to think, to create. If we are open to it we expand our horizons. If we are closed then stagnation sets in.

Through nurturing an internal stillness we are able to receive God's grace. Prayer and meditation provide the key.

Reflection: God's Grace

+ **Walking Light**

Spirituality is developed through the decision to care for ourselves and others. That in turn helps us acknowledge God's presence in our lives. Then we can begin to gain a degree of comfort between what we understand and what is difficult to accept.

+ **Personal Path**

Write about an effective way you connect to God.

To keep a lamp burning,
we have to keep putting oil into it.

—Mother Teresa

Stop Signs

It is said in Latin America that a stop sign is more of a suggestion than a command! At times the drivers in our neighborhood have adopted the south-of-the-border philosophy. I am cautious at 5:30 AM when we approach intersections. The alternative is a recipe for disaster.

Most of us are not enthusiastic about some of the rules that govern our daily life. However, it is because of such guidelines we have a more peaceful coexistence instead of chaos.

As walkers we have different responsibilities. The law requires drivers to follow such posted directions as a stop sign. However, it is when everyone pays attention that an endeavor goes successfully.

Reflection: Guidelines

+ **Walking Light**

Guidelines foster growth. As we move through life some guidelines may need to be "updated." Other personal rules tend to remain constant, for they benefit the common good. We need to be able to make that distinction.

+ **Personal Path**

Identify in your journal personal guidelines that have been helpful. These can be drawn from your home life, professional activities, or a special relationship.

Learn the three "R's", Respect for self,
Respect for others and
Responsibility for all your actions.

—Dalai Lama

Announcements

Often "they" are like mushrooms that seem to pop up overnight. "They" might be a "For Sale" sign, a six-foot wooden stork proclaiming the newest addition to a family, or an American flag. All of these represent something significant to the home's residents.

Self-talk is an internal announcement. Silently it can affirm or condemn. What you say to yourself impacts the quality of each day.

Eventually the announcement signs that Molly, Calvin, and I walk by disappear. The changes that prompted the placement of these signs do not vanish. If the theme of your self-talk is constructive, you can build a better tomorrow. If not, life can become overwhelming.

Reflection: Self-Esteem

+ **Walking Light**

Healthy self-esteem is an "inside job." If negative internal statements intrude in daily life, use them as a springboard towards constructive and nurturing alternatives. What you say about yourself is what you project to the world around you.

+ **Personal Path**

In your journal write three positive comments others say about you. Next write three traits about yourself that you like. Be aware of these.

Nobody knows what's in him until he tries to pull it out.

—Ernest Hemingway

Breather

In the predawn stillness we approached a familiar stop sign. This morning there was something different about the scene. Leaning against the support post was a child's bicycle. How appropriate it seemed to have such a toy resting against this traffic sign. Play had ceased for the day. The child and bike are at rest.

We need to stop and catch our breath. Exhaustion leads to emptiness. Pausing for a while allows us to renew our physical, emotional, and spiritual lives.

The bicycle will soon be retrieved. Playtime will continue. When we are refreshed it allows us to live and love to our best ability.

Reflection: Rest

✦ Walking Light

Resting is about an activity that refreshes both body and spirit. Essentially it is taking a time-out for yourself without feeling guilty. This is not about how much time but the quality of your effort to renew.

✦ Personal Path

Record times when you felt rested. Were they planned or spur of the moment?

Whatever does not rest, will not endure.

—Ovid

Walking

The pattern is familiar. Placing one foot or paw in front of the other and repeating this many times is how we make our rounds. The pace may be leisurely, but it is purposeful. The journey is completed because we kept walking.

When we approach each day with a purpose, goals are achieved. Ideas become reality. If the focus is exclusively on the past, moving forward becomes more difficult.

Our life's direction is determined through our actions. A steady pace, a defined direction, and a belief in your abilities combine to achieve goals.

Reflection: Assertiveness

+ Walking Light

In life there is movement. Assertiveness channels that movement into you, defining what is important. In doing so you are establishing how you wish to live. Finally, that improves the quality of interactions.

+ Personal Path

Journaling is an assertive action. It records honestly how you experience life. Write about a time when you acted on a strong belief.

The basic difference between being assertive and being aggressive is how our words and behaviors affect the rights and well-being of others.

—*Sharon Anthony Bower*

Tailwind

Stepping out of the front door this morning I noticed how windy it had become overnight. Calvin, Molly, and I initially head west into our neighborhood. A strong ocean breeze was coming into our backs. A plastic cup rattled by, loose paper was wrapped around a signpost, and the dogs' fur was ruffled. Nature was encouraging everything including us to move along.

Encouragement keeps us motivated. The helping words and hands of others nurture our confidence. At times, others can see our possibilities when our view is clouded. Ultimately we reach our goal.

On the return path home we walked back into the same wind. The dogs and I were looking forward to breakfast. Working together we all achieve this reward.

Reflection: Encouragement

+ **Walking Light**

Encouragement is a caring gift. It is seeing the potential in others. It is fostering belief in others when they are unable to see it in themselves. Encouragement is acknowledging God's belief in all of us.

+ **Personal Path**

Write about a time when you worked through a trying situation. How important was the encouragement you received?

A word of encouragement during a failure is worth more than an hour of praise after success.

—Anonymous

Different Sounds

The neighborhood is dark two of the three times we walk. Yet in that darkness there are distinct differences. The sounds of morning are that of an awakening world. There is a hushed gentleness. In the evening, even late, the variety and frequency of the ambient noise is more intense. The lives of commerce and nature change as the day unfolds.

Each day is different in subtle and sometimes dramatic ways. We adapt to the new day from the time we rise in the morning to "lights out" many hours later. We do this without giving it much thought. This coping process helps define our strengths.

I am not certain what Molly and Calvin hear or how they interpret it. They certainly react to the commotion of traffic or the sound of a distant feline. What I do know is that at the end of each walk we all have learned from the experiences. This adds to our coping skills for the next outing.

Reflection: Coping

+ **Walking Light**

When the familiar changes, we can either cope or resist. In adapting we have the opportunity to stretch known boundaries and grow. For certain we did this every day in school. We continue to do the same each new morning.

+ **Personal Path**

Write about a time when you moved. How did you meet the challenges of that event?

Problems are not the problem; coping is the problem.

—Virginia Satir

Arbor Day

For years every Arbor Day children were given a pencil-thick twig to plant. It was a free tree! Years ago when we began to walk around our neighborhood a young student planted several of these in the side-yard of the family house. It seems like just yesterday they were only knee high; now we can pause in the shade of these trees.

Ignoring little distractions or irritations in life can evolve into undesirable results. Depression, chemical dependency, or abusive behaviors are quite subtle at the beginning. Eventually they absorb more energy and become a dominant feature in our lifestyle.

Today these large side yard trees now form a distinct part of the landscape. It is our responsibility to pay attention to those parts of life that can ultimately impact the quality of living.

Reflection: Paying Attention

◆ Walking Light
Paying attention to the present has many benefits. Experiencing the moment helps you build a healthier tomorrow. When we do this it also provides a time to modify problematic patterns.

◆ Personal Path
Write about a small difference you noticed today in yourself, your partner, or a child.

You can become blind by seeing each day as a similar one. Each day is a different one, each day brings a miracle of its own. It's just a matter of paying attention to this miracle.

—Paulo Coelho

Breezes

The ocean breezes almost constantly are rustling through the palm trees along our walk. I can't see the wind, but its presence is readily noticeable. The wind moves seeds and pollen to new places for life to begin again.

We have an unseen inner wind. It is known by many names—spirit and soul are just two. It moves us to grow, create, and endure. When our physical forms become still, this unseen wind carries us into a new life in eternity.

Be aware of the spirit within you. By doing so you are honoring its Creator and you.

Reflection: Spirituality

✦ Walking Light
The "breeze" of God's spirit is always moving inside of us. Sometimes it is quite soft, almost a whisper, and other times it is strong and passionate. It manifests itself through our kind thoughts and deeds.

✦ Personal Path
Recall a prayer from your childhood. Say it with the sincerity of a child. Write about how this felt both then and now.

Sometimes people get the mistaken notion that spirituality is a separate department of life, the penthouse of existence. But rightly understood, it is a vital awareness that pervades all realms of our being.

—David Steindl-Rast

Green Branch

Molly, Calvin, and I often are walking around or over fallen palm branches. Yesterday a bright green one fell just ahead of us, hitting the pavement with a familiar thud. Then something unexpected happened. In a few seconds the "branch" got up, shook itself off, and ran into the nearby bushes. It wasn't a branch at all but a bright green iguana! The fall certainly stunned the creature but did not seem to have a lasting impact.

In life we stumble and fall. Setbacks come from many directions. The challenge is to pick ourselves up and continue life. The resilience to keep moving comes from within you. The alternative is to give up.

The iguana quickly returned to its natural habitat. We also need to continue when we experience a setback. The wisdom we can gain from such an event cannot be acquired in any other manner.

Reflection: Resilience

♦ Walking Light

Resilience is found in both success and failure. Lessons are in each. Learning from them is optional. It is in understanding your part in either outcome that the experience is optimized

♦ Personal Path

Rebounding after a difficulty is important. In your journal, write about recovering from a challenging time or event.

Our greatest glory is not in never falling but in rising every time we fall.

—Confucius

Signs

Two weeks after I picked Calvin up from the Sheltie Rescue, he decided to go for a walk—by himself! What became evident was that he ran considerably faster than I. As the distance grew we both shared a common emotion—fear. The busy streets that border our neighborhood presented a peril I did not want to think about.

The pursuit of Calvin was not going well. I needed help. I posted signs around the area, asking for assistance. Several people called and even tried to catch him but were unsuccessful. The next day I picked up a remorseful Calvin at the county animal shelter.

Asking for help can be difficult. I went as far as I could in finding Calvin, but I realized it was not possible alone. In life we are responsible to do the best we can. Asking for help allows us to grow even further. In the end it takes strength to reach out. We need to acknowledge our limits, and when necessary, be open to assistance in expanding them.

Reflection: Helping

♦ Walking Light

To ask for help is about growth. Helping another is about coopera-tion and caring. Both require a transition from thinking into action.

♦ Personal Path

When have you helped someone or been helped? Looking back over the past few days write about being of assistance to someone. Who changed as a result of this action?

In about the same degree as you are helpful,
you will be happy.

—Karl Reiland

Six Cents

Just in front of us on the pavement were two coins—a nickel and a penny. It was not a fortune but it was there for the finder. I put them in my pocket eventually, to be added to a can of accumulated coins at home and hopefully put to good use.

To have a healthy life requires finding hope. With hope, ideas flow into actions and actions into accomplishments. Hope is a self-renewing resource.

Molly, Calvin, and I continued our walk not paying much attention to the discarded change I picked up. In the small effort it took to retrieve the six cents a little hope was generated. Fostering hope creates the future.

Reflection: Hope

♦ Walking Light

Hope gives meaning to our lives. Yet incorporating it into our lives requires effort. Such effort is based on belief in ourselves and the path we choose to follow.

♦ Personal Path

Write about a specific hope you have for your personal future. What is a preliminary step you can take today to turn that hope into a reality?

Once you choose hope, anything is possible.

—Christopher Reeve

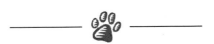

Dog Walking Journal

The journaling (Personal Path) exercise is one way to explore your own insights. If journaling is new to you, the following may be helpful.

Five Keys to "the Personal Experience"

Key One: Use of the senses—to hear, to see, to touch, to smell, to taste. For example, one may see a beautiful sunrise while another at the same time may be more impressed by the silence of the early morning. Both observations reflect the uniqueness of each individual's experience. There is no right or wrong to what is perceived.

Key Two: Emotional awareness. Once your senses note something of interest, be aware of your feelings. Sadness, humor, poignancy, joy, and so forth are emotional reactions. Your emotional reaction can be subtle and even delayed a bit, but it is still there. Try to "name" the emotional impact. Remember, whatever the feeling, it is your truth.

Key Three: Curiosity. It may be difficult to determine which came first— an emotional reaction to something or cognitive interest. The essential factor here is being in the "now." This allows you to absorb what is happening around you at the very moment. Disconnecting from outside (electronic) interference reduces distractions.

Key Four: Discover the meaning. For example, if you see someone's generosity, what does it remind you about yourself? What values are found as a result of the experience? Being aware of your own core beliefs and principles is essential. It may be helpful to look at the various topics presented in *Dog Walking* to stimulate your own list.

Key Five: Individuality. Journaling can be in any style you wish. Random thoughts, a phrase, a word or two, poetry, a formal narrative, even a sketch. An important factor in journaling is honesty. Remember, it is essentially a reflection of yourself and for your eyes only. Write whenever you wish. Days or even weeks may go by between reading a story and making a written comment. That is OK.

The effort it takes to journal nourishes you. You are worth the effort.

The following pages can provide a beginning space for your journaling. This can be further expanded in a notebook or computer. The sequence of the topics is the same as in the book.

Story: **Sheepless**

Theme: **Playtime**

I enjoy doing:

Story: **The Lizard Chaser and Mr. Cool**

Theme: **Nurturing Relationships**

I encouraged someone when:

_____

_____

_____

_____

_____

_____

_____

_____

_____

_____

_____

_____

_____

_____

_____

_____

_____

_____

_____

_____

_____

Story: **Cloud Topper**

Theme: **Small Kindnesses**

What thoughtful behavior recently happened to me?

Story: **Distance**

Theme: **Balance**

When I need to "recharge," I:

_____

_____

_____

_____

_____

_____

_____

_____

_____

_____

_____

_____

_____

_____

_____

_____

_____

_____

_____

_____

_____

_____

_____

_____

Story: **Bulk Trash Pickup**

Theme: **Heritage**

I admire this quality about one of my family members:

_____

_____

_____

_____

_____

_____

_____

_____

_____

_____

_____

_____

_____

_____

_____

_____

_____

_____

_____

_____

_____

Story: **Stains**

Theme: **Perspective**

What recently changed my mind about a person, place, or philosophy?

Story: **Taxi**

Theme: **Compassion**

When did I donate something for a cause and what was it?

_____

_____

_____

_____

_____

_____

_____

_____

_____

_____

_____

_____

_____

_____

_____

_____

_____

_____

_____

_____

Story: **Floating Lights**

Theme: **Emotional Well-Being**

I nurture myself by:

_____

_____

_____

_____

_____

_____

_____

_____

_____

_____

_____

_____

_____

_____

_____

_____

_____

_____

_____

_____

Story: **Sidewalk Patterns**

Theme: **Core Values**

An important lesson I learned in childhood that I use today is:

Story: **Fast Walks**

Theme: **Possibilities**

Each new day has possibilities for growth because I:

_____

_____

_____

_____

_____

_____

_____

_____

_____

_____

_____

_____

_____

_____

_____

_____

_____

_____

_____

_____

_____

_____

Story: **Senses**

Theme: **Awareness**

My sense of (*one of your five senses—hearing, touch, sight, smell, taste*)
_____ **stirs in me the feeling of:**

Story: **Half-Staffed**

Theme: **Connectedness**

Who was my favorite teacher in school and why?

Story: **Things That Go Bump in the Night**

Theme: **Courage**

I work hard on achieving:

Story: **Seamless**

Theme: **Confidence**

I am good at:

Story: **And Then There Were Three—Almost**

Theme: **Dreams**

My dream in life is to:

_____

_____

_____

_____

_____

_____

_____

_____

_____

_____

_____

_____

_____

_____

_____

_____

_____

_____

_____

_____

_____

_____

_____

_____

Story: **Colors**

Theme: **Transitions**

When plans change I:

Story: **Wet Feet**

Theme: **Uniqueness**

It is uncomfortable for me to express:

Story: **Bells and Whistles**

Theme: **Simplicity**

A simple habit I enjoy doing each day is:

_____

_____

_____

_____

_____

_____

_____

_____

_____

_____

_____

_____

_____

_____

_____

_____

_____

_____

_____

_____

Story: **Blink**

Theme: **Trust**

The person I trust most is:

_____

_____

_____

_____

_____

_____

_____

_____

_____

_____

_____

_____

_____

_____

_____

_____

_____

_____

_____

_____

Story: **Two Trees**

Theme: **True Wealth**

What do I value most in life?

_____

_____

_____

_____

_____

_____

_____

_____

_____

_____

_____

_____

_____

_____

_____

_____

_____

_____

_____

_____

_____

Story: **Wind Chimes**

Theme: **Potential**

I need_____ to achieve my goals.
When can I begin?"

_____

_____

_____

_____

_____

_____

_____

_____

_____

_____

_____

_____

_____

_____

_____

_____

_____

_____

_____

Story: **A Familiar Song**

Theme: **Prayer**

Prayer helps me when:

Story: **Strays**

Theme: **Healthy Choices**

I benefit when I choose to:

_____

_____

_____

_____

_____

_____

_____

_____

_____

_____

_____

_____

_____

_____

_____

_____

_____

_____

_____

_____

_____

Story: **Moving Day**

Theme: **Optimism**

Tomorrow I want to:

_____

_____

_____

_____

_____

_____

_____

_____

_____

_____

_____

_____

_____

_____

_____

_____

_____

_____

_____

_____

Story: **Daylight**

Theme: **Getting Unstuck**

A habit I changed was:

_____

_____

_____

_____

_____

_____

_____

_____

_____

_____

_____

_____

_____

_____

_____

_____

_____

_____

_____

_____

Story: **Dog Ears**

Theme: **Cooperation**

I volunteered to:

_____

_____

_____

_____

_____

_____

_____

_____

_____

_____

_____

_____

_____

_____

_____

_____

_____

_____

_____

_____

_____

_____

Story: **Going Outside**

Theme: **Patience**

I am very tolerant about:

_____

_____

_____

_____

_____

_____

_____

_____

_____

_____

_____

_____

_____

_____

_____

_____

_____

_____

_____

_____

_____

_____

Story: **Night**

Theme: **Living Through Loss**

A loss in my life was:

_____

_____

_____

_____

_____

_____

_____

_____

_____

_____

_____

_____

_____

_____

_____

_____

_____

_____

_____

_____

Story: **Dry**

Theme: **Conservation**

I do my part in helping to preserve the natural environment by:

Story: **Office Neighborhood Friend**

Theme: **Joy**

The last time I laughed out loud was when:

_____

_____

_____

_____

_____

_____

_____

_____

_____

_____

_____

_____

_____

_____

_____

_____

_____

_____

_____

_____

_____

Story: **Trees On Wheels**

Theme: **Family**

What is an important tradition in my family?

_____

_____

_____

_____

_____

_____

_____

_____

_____

_____

_____

_____

_____

_____

_____

_____

_____

_____

_____

_____

_____

Story: **Curbside**

Theme: **Gratitude**

I express appreciation by:

Story: **The Biscuit Lady**

Theme: **Giving**

Giving to me means:

_____

_____

_____

_____

_____

_____

_____

_____

_____

_____

_____

_____

_____

_____

_____

_____

_____

_____

_____

_____

_____

_____

_____

Story: **Hold On Tight**

Theme: **Problem Solving**

I solve problems by:

_____

_____

_____

_____

_____

_____

_____

_____

_____

_____

_____

_____

_____

_____

_____

_____

_____

_____

_____

_____

Story: **Passages**

Theme: **Identity**

What cause is important to you?

What corporate logo(s) are on clothes that you wear?

Which of the above reflects your identity and why?

Story: **Shooting Stars**

Theme: **Prioritizing**

It is easier to begin a task when:

Story: **Runner**

Theme: **Exercise**

Physical exercise to me is:

Story: **Stars in Puddles**

Theme: **Mourning**

Describe what it means to survive a loss:

_____

_____

_____

_____

_____

_____

_____

_____

_____

_____

_____

_____

_____

_____

_____

_____

_____

_____

_____

_____

_____

_____

Story: **Mailbox**

Theme: **God's Grace**

I recognize God's presence in my life when:

_____

_____

_____

_____

_____

_____

_____

_____

_____

_____

_____

_____

_____

_____

_____

_____

_____

_____

_____

_____

_____

_____

Story: **Stop Signs**

Theme: **Guidelines**

A good rule for me to follow in life is:

_____

_____

_____

_____

_____

_____

_____

_____

_____

_____

_____

_____

_____

_____

_____

_____

_____

_____

Story: **Announcements**

Theme: **Self-Esteem**

Write about your top three strengths:

Story: **Breather**

Theme: **Rest**

When I take a time-out I like to:

_____

_____

_____

_____

_____

_____

_____

_____

_____

_____

_____

_____

_____

_____

_____

_____

_____

_____

_____

_____

_____

_____

Story: **Walking**

Theme: **Assertiveness**

Describe a time when I stood up for what I believed when:

_____

_____

_____

_____

_____

_____

_____

_____

_____

_____

_____

_____

_____

_____

_____

_____

_____

_____

_____

Story: **Tailwind**

Theme: **Encouragement**

I have received support when:

_____

_____

_____

_____

_____

_____

_____

_____

_____

_____

_____

_____

_____

_____

_____

_____

_____

_____

_____

_____

_____

Story: **Different Sounds**

Theme: **Coping**

Adapting to change is easier because I:

Story: **Arbor Day**

Theme: **Paying Attention**

What is different about me today?

_____

_____

_____

_____

_____

_____

_____

_____

_____

_____

_____

_____

_____

_____

_____

_____

_____

_____

_____

_____

_____

Story: **Breezes**

Theme: **Spirituality**

How do I nurture my connection with God?

Story: **Green Branch**

Theme: **Resilience**

Recovering from a disappointment is important because:

Story: **Signs**

Theme: **Helping**

When is it difficult to help someone?

Story: **Six Cents**

Theme: **Hope**

I am most hopeful for:

_____

_____

_____

_____

_____

_____

_____

_____

_____

_____

_____

_____

_____

_____

_____

_____

_____

_____

_____

_____

_____

_____

About the Author

John is a licensed psychotherapist and has been in private practice for more than twenty-five years in Fort Lauderdale, Florida. His therapy with couples, individuals, and families focuses on communication and stress-related problems. When traumatic events occur in the workplace impacting employees, John provides on-site clinical support. He also conducts workshops on grief, relationships, and life coping skills.

John holds a B.S. degree from the University of Cincinnati. He completed graduate studies in pastoral ministry at Miami's St. Thomas University with additional work in counseling psychology. He is a state-licensed mental health counselor. He is nationally certified in psychotherapy, grief, and trauma.

John's relationship with the canine world began when he and his twin brother, Tom, came home from the hospital. They were cautiously greeted by their parents' Collie, Buster. Through the years, his life has been enriched by the companionship of dogs.

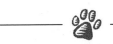